MEDICAL HISTORY

medical history

personal records journal

This journal belongs to: ______________________________

Disclaimer: This journal is ***not*** *intended to diagnose or treat anything. You should consult a doctor before using this journal. No liability will be accepted for any use or misuse. You use at your own risk and accept all liability.*

MEDICAL HISTORY

PERSONAL RECORDS JOURNAL

MEDICAL HISTORY

JAV PUBLISHING

Printed in the United Stated of America

*Disclaimer: This journal is **not** intended to diagnose or treat anything. You should consult a doctor before using this journal. No liability will be accepted for any use or misuse. You use at your own risk and accept all liability.*

ISBN-10: 0615604552
ISBN-13: 978-0615604558

PERSONAL DATA

NAME:

ADDRESS:

CITY: STATE: ZIP:

TELEPHONE NUMBER:

WORK NUMBER:

BIRTH DATE:

SOCIAL SECURITY NUMBER:

BLOOD TYPE: ETHNIC BACKGROUND:

HEIGHT: WEIGHT:

SOCIAL SECURITY NUMBER:

ALLERGIES:

SPECIFIC MEDICAL NEEDS:

ORGAN DONOR: YES NO

POWER OF ATTORNEY:

LIVING WILL: YES NO

PRIMARY CARE PHYSICIAN

NAME:

ADDRESS:

CITY: STATE: ZIP:

TELEPHONE NUMBER:

PREFERRED HOSPITAL:

NOTES:

SPOUSE'S DATA

NAME:

ADDRESS:

CITY: STATE: ZIP:

TELEPHONE NUMBER:

WORK NUMBER:

BIRTH DATE:

SOCIAL SECURITY NUMBER:

BLOOD TYPE: ETHNIC BACKGROUND:

HEIGHT: WEIGHT:

SOCIAL SECURITY NUMBER:

ALLERGIES:

SPECIFIC MEDICAL NEEDS:

ORGAN DONOR: YES NO

POWER OF ATTORNEY:

LIVING WILL: YES NO

PRIMARY CARE PHYSICIAN

NAME:

ADDRESS:

CITY: STATE: ZIP:

TELEPHONE NUMBER:

PREFERRED HOSPITAL:

NOTES:

CHILD'S DATA

NAME:

ADDRESS:

CITY: STATE: ZIP:

TELEPHONE NUMBER:

WORK NUMBER:

BIRTH DATE:

SOCIAL SECURITY NUMBER:

BLOOD TYPE: ETHNIC BACKGROUND:

HEIGHT: WEIGHT:

SOCIAL SECURITY NUMBER:

ALLERGIES:

SPECIFIC MEDICAL NEEDS:

ORGAN DONOR: YES NO

POWER OF ATTORNEY:

LIVING WILL: YES NO

PRIMARY CARE PHYSICIAN

NAME:

ADDRESS:

CITY: STATE: ZIP:

TELEPHONE NUMBER:

PREFERRED HOSPITAL:

NOTES:

CHILD'S DATA

NAME:

ADDRESS:

CITY: STATE: ZIP:

TELEPHONE NUMBER:

WORK NUMBER:

BIRTH DATE:

SOCIAL SECURITY NUMBER:

BLOOD TYPE: ETHNIC BACKGROUND:

HEIGHT: WEIGHT:

SOCIAL SECURITY NUMBER:

ALLERGIES:

SPECIFIC MEDICAL NEEDS:

ORGAN DONOR: YES NO

POWER OF ATTORNEY:

LIVING WILL: YES NO

PRIMARY CARE PHYSICIAN

NAME:

ADDRESS:

CITY: STATE: ZIP:

TELEPHONE NUMBER:

PREFERRED HOSPITAL:

NOTES:

CHILD'S DATA

NAME:

ADDRESS:

CITY: STATE: ZIP:

TELEPHONE NUMBER:

WORK NUMBER:

BIRTH DATE:

SOCIAL SECURITY NUMBER:

BLOOD TYPE: ETHNIC BACKGROUND:

HEIGHT: WEIGHT:

SOCIAL SECURITY NUMBER:

ALLERGIES:

SPECIFIC MEDICAL NEEDS:

ORGAN DONOR: YES NO

POWER OF ATTORNEY:

LIVING WILL: YES NO

PRIMARY CARE PHYSICIAN

NAME:

ADDRESS:

CITY: STATE: ZIP:

TELEPHONE NUMBER:

PREFERRED HOSPITAL:

NOTES:

CHILD'S DATA

NAME:

ADDRESS:

CITY: STATE: ZIP:

TELEPHONE NUMBER:

WORK NUMBER:

BIRTH DATE:

SOCIAL SECURITY NUMBER:

BLOOD TYPE: ETHNIC BACKGROUND:

HEIGHT: WEIGHT:

SOCIAL SECURITY NUMBER:

ALLERGIES:

SPECIFIC MEDICAL NEEDS:

ORGAN DONOR: YES NO

POWER OF ATTORNEY:

LIVING WILL: YES NO

PRIMARY CARE PHYSICIAN

NAME:

ADDRESS:

CITY: STATE: ZIP:

TELEPHONE NUMBER:

PREFERRED HOSPITAL:

NOTES:

EMERGENCY CONTACTS

NAME: RELATIONSHIP:
ADDRESS:
CITY: STATE: ZIP:
HOME NUMBER:
CELL NUMBER:
WORK NUMBER:

NAME: RELATIONSHIP:
ADDRESS:
CITY: STATE: ZIP:
HOME NUMBER:
CELL NUMBER:
WORK NUMBER:

NAME: RELATIONSHIP:
ADDRESS:
CITY: STATE: ZIP:
HOME NUMBER:
CELL NUMBER:
WORK NUMBER:

NAME: RELATIONSHIP:
ADDRESS:
CITY: STATE: ZIP:
HOME NUMBER:
CELL NUMBER:
WORK NUMBER:

FATHER'S FULL NAME:
MOTHER'S FULL NAME:
YOUR MAIDEN NAME:
OTHER NAMES USED:

SPOUSE'S EMERGENCY CONTACTS

NAME: RELATIONSHIP:
ADDRESS:
CITY: STATE: ZIP:
HOME NUMBER:
CELL NUMBER:
WORK NUMBER:

NAME: RELATIONSHIP:
ADDRESS:
CITY: STATE: ZIP:
HOME NUMBER:
CELL NUMBER:
WORK NUMBER:

NAME: RELATIONSHIP:
ADDRESS:
CITY: STATE: ZIP:
HOME NUMBER:
CELL NUMBER:
WORK NUMBER:

NAME: RELATIONSHIP:
ADDRESS:
CITY: STATE: ZIP:
HOME NUMBER:
CELL NUMBER:
WORK NUMBER:

FATHER'S FULL NAME:
MOTHER'S FULL NAME:
YOUR MAIDEN NAME:
OTHER NAMES USED:

HEALTHCARE INSURANCE INFORMATION

PRIMARY HEALTHCARE:

POLICY OWNER: POLICY NO:

PAYER ID:

GROUP NAME: GROUP NO:

TELEPHONE NUMBER:

FAX NUMBER:

EFFECTIVE DATE:

NOTES:

SECONDARY HEALTHCARE:

POLICY OWNER: POLICY NO:

PAYER ID:

GROUP NAME: GROUP NO:

TELEPHONE NUMBER:

FAX NUMBER:

EFFECTIVE DATE:

NOTES:

MEDICARE / MEDICAID

POLICY NUMBER:

EFFECTIVE DATE:

TELEPHONE NUMBER:

FAX NUMBER:

NOTES:

PHYISCIAN'S NAME:

TELEPHONE NUMBER:

FAX NUMBER:

ADDRESS:

CITY: STATE: ZIP:

DENTAL INSURANCE PROVIDER

DENTAL PROVIDER:

POLICY OWNER: POLICY NO:

PAYER ID:

GROUP NAME: GROUP NO:

TELEPHONE NUMBER:

FAX NUMBER:

EFFECTIVE DATE:

NOTES:

SECONDARY DENTAL PROVIDER:

POLICY OWNER: POLICY NO:

PAYER ID:

GROUP NAME: GROUP NO:

TELEPHONE NUMBER:

FAX NUMBER:

EFFECTIVE DATE:

NOTES:

DENTIST NAME:

TELEPHONE NUMBER:

FAX NUMBER:

ADDRESS:

CITY: STATE: ZIP:

PATIENT SINCE:

NOTES:

VISION INSURANCE PROVIDER

VISION PROVIDER:

POLICY OWNER: POLICY NO:

PAYER ID:

GROUP NAME: GROUP NO:

TELEPHONE NUMBER:

FAX NUMBER:

EFFECTIVE DATE:

NOTES:

SECONDARY VISION PROVIDER:

POLICY OWNER: POLICY NO:

PAYER ID:

GROUP NAME: GROUP NO:

TELEPHONE NUMBER:

FAX NUMBER:

EFFECTIVE DATE:

NOTES:

DENTIST NAME:

TELEPHONE NUMBER:

FAX NUMBER:

ADDRESS:

CITY: STATE: ZIP:

PATIENT SINCE:

NOTES:

OTHER INFORMATION

LIFE INSURANCE:

POLICY OWNER:

POLICY NUMBER:

TELEPHONE NUMBER:

CHURCH NAME:

PASTOR:

TELEPHONE NUMBER:

ADDRESS:

CITY: STATE: ZIP:

FUNERAL HOME NAME:

TELEPHONE NUMBER:

ADDRESS:

CITY: STATE: ZIP:

FUNERAL PAID: YES NO

NOTE:

CEMETERY NAME:

TELEPHONE NUMBER:

ADDRESS:

CITY: STATE: ZIP:

NOTE:

ATTORNEY:

TELEPHONE NUMBER:

ADDRESS:

CITY: STATE: ZIP:

TELEPHONE NUMBER:

YOUR MEDICAL HISTORY

YOUR FULL NAME:

*Disclaimer: This journal is **not** intended to diagnose or treat anything. You should consult a doctor before using this journal. No liability will be accepted for any use or misuse. You use at your own risk and accept all liability.*

Condition	Age at Onset	Treatment	Result
Alzheimer's Disease			
Allergic Rhinitis (Hay fever)			
Anemia			
Anesthesia Problem			
Arthritis			
Asthma			
Birth Defects			
Bleeding Problem			
Cancer, Breast			
Cancer, Colon			
Cancer, Lung			
Cancer, Melanoma			
Cancer, Prostate			
Cancer, Skin			
Cancer, Ovarian			
Cancer (other)			
Depression			
Diabetes, Type 1			
Diabetes, Type 2			
Epilepsy (seizures)			
Eye Conditions			
Glaucoma			
Hearing Problems			
Heart Disease (Coronary Artery or Heart Attack)			
High Cholesterol			

Condition	Age at Onset	Treatment	Result
High Blood Pressure			
Kidney Diseases			
Lupus			
Mental Retardation			
Migraine Headaches			
Miscarriage			
Osteoarthritis			
Osteoporosis			
Rheumatoid Arthritis			
Stroke			
Thyroid Disorders			
Tuberculosis			
Ulcer			
Other:			

OTHER FACTORS

Condition	Age at Onset	Treatment	Result
Alcoholism			
Drug Use			
Obesity			
Smoking			

LIST OF ANY HOSPITALIZATIONS

HOSPITAL: DATE:

REASON:

RESULT:

HOSPITAL: DATE:

REASON:

RESULT:

*Disclaimer: This journal is **not** intended to diagnose or treat anything. You should consult a doctor before using this journal. No liability will be accepted for any use or misuse. You use at your own risk and accept all liability.*

NOTES

*Disclaimer: This journal is **not** intended to diagnose or treat anything. You should consult a doctor before using this journal. No liability will be accepted for any use or misuse. You use at your own risk and accept all liability.*

FATHER MEDICAL HISTORY

FULL NAME:

*Disclaimer: This journal is **not** intended to diagnose or treat anything. You should consult a doctor before using this journal. No liability will be accepted for any use or misuse. You use at your own risk and accept all liability.*

Condition	Age at Onset	Treatment	Result
Alzheimer's Disease			
Allergic Rhinitis (Hay fever)			
Anemia			
Anesthesia Problem			
Arthritis			
Asthma			
Birth Defects			
Bleeding Problem			
Cancer, Breast			
Cancer, Colon			
Cancer, Lung			
Cancer, Melanoma			
Cancer, Prostate			
Cancer, Skin			
Cancer, Ovarian			
Cancer (other)			
Depression			
Diabetes, Type 1			
Diabetes, Type 2			
Epilepsy (seizures)			
Eye Conditions			
Glaucoma			
Hearing Problems			
Heart Disease (Coronary Artery or Heart Attack)			
High Cholesterol			

Condition	Age at Onset	Treatment	Result
High Blood Pressure			
Kidney Diseases			
Lupus			
Mental Retardation			
Migraine Headaches			
Miscarriage			
Osteoarthritis			
Osteoporosis			
Rheumatoid Arthritis			
Stroke			
Thyroid Disorders			
Tuberculosis			
Ulcer			
Other:			

OTHER FACTORS

Condition	Age at Onset	Treatment	Result
Alcoholism			
Drug Use			
Obesity			
Smoking			

LIST OF ANY HOSPITALIZATIONS

HOSPITAL: DATE:

REASON:

RESULT:

HOSPITAL: DATE:

REASON:

RESULT:

*Disclaimer: This journal is **not** intended to diagnose or treat anything. You should consult a doctor before using this journal. No liability will be accepted for any use or misuse. You use at your own risk and accept all liability.*

NOTES

*Disclaimer: This journal is **not** intended to diagnose or treat anything. You should consult a doctor before using this journal. No liability will be accepted for any use or misuse. You use at your own risk and accept all liability.*

MOTHER MEDICAL HISTORY

FULL NAME:

*Disclaimer: This journal is **not** intended to diagnose or treat anything. You should consult a doctor before using this journal. No liability will be accepted for any use or misuse. You use at your own risk and accept all liability.*

Condition	Age at Onset	Treatment	Result
Alzheimer's Disease			
Allergic Rhinitis (Hay fever)			
Anemia			
Anesthesia Problem			
Arthritis			
Asthma			
Birth Defects			
Bleeding Problem			
Cancer, Breast			
Cancer, Colon			
Cancer, Lung			
Cancer, Melanoma			
Cancer, Prostate			
Cancer, Skin			
Cancer, Ovarian			
Cancer (other)			
Depression			
Diabetes, Type 1			
Diabetes, Type 2			
Epilepsy (seizures)			
Eye Conditions			
Glaucoma			
Hearing Problems			
Heart Disease (Coronary Artery or Heart Attack)			
High Cholesterol			

Condition	Age at Onset	Treatment	Result
High Blood Pressure			
Kidney Diseases			
Lupus			
Mental Retardation			
Migraine Headaches			
Miscarriage			
Osteoarthritis			
Osteoporosis			
Rheumatoid Arthritis			
Stroke			
Thyroid Disorders			
Tuberculosis			
Ulcer			
Other:			

OTHER FACTORS

Condition	Age at Onset	Treatment	Result
Alcoholism			
Drug Use			
Obesity			
Smoking			

LIST OF ANY HOSPITALIZATIONS

HOSPITAL: DATE:

REASON:

RESULT:

HOSPITAL: DATE:

REASON:

RESULT:

*Disclaimer: This journal is **not** intended to diagnose or treat anything. You should consult a doctor before using this journal. No liability will be accepted for any use or misuse. You use at your own risk and accept all liability.*

NOTES

*Disclaimer: This journal is **not** intended to diagnose or treat anything. You should consult a doctor before using this journal. No liability will be accepted for any use or misuse. You use at your own risk and accept all liability.*

BROTHER OR SISTER MEDICAL HISTORY

FULL NAME:

*Disclaimer: This journal is **not** intended to diagnose or treat anything. You should consult a doctor before using this journal. No liability will be accepted for any use or misuse. You use at your own risk and accept all liability.*

Condition	Age at Onset	Treatment	Result
Alzheimer's Disease			
Allergic Rhinitis (Hay fever)			
Anemia			
Anesthesia Problem			
Arthritis			
Asthma			
Birth Defects			
Bleeding Problem			
Cancer, Breast			
Cancer, Colon			
Cancer, Lung			
Cancer, Melanoma			
Cancer, Prostate			
Cancer, Skin			
Cancer, Ovarian			
Cancer (other)			
Depression			
Diabetes, Type 1			
Diabetes, Type 2			
Epilepsy (seizures)			
Eye Conditions			
Glaucoma			
Hearing Problems			
Heart Disease (Coronary Artery or Heart Attack)			
High Cholesterol			

Condition	Age at Onset	Treatment	Result
High Blood Pressure			
Kidney Diseases			
Lupus			
Mental Retardation			
Migraine Headaches			
Miscarriage			
Osteoarthritis			
Osteoporosis			
Rheumatoid Arthritis			
Stroke			
Thyroid Disorders			
Tuberculosis			
Ulcer			
Other:			

OTHER FACTORS

Condition	Age at Onset	Treatment	Result
Alcoholism			
Drug Use			
Obesity			
Smoking			

LIST OF ANY HOSPITALIZATIONS

HOSPITAL: DATE:

REASON:

RESULT:

HOSPITAL: DATE:

REASON:

RESULT:

*Disclaimer: This journal is **not** intended to diagnose or treat anything. You should consult a doctor before using this journal. No liability will be accepted for any use or misuse. You use at your own risk and accept all liability.*

NOTES

*Disclaimer: This journal is **not** intended to diagnose or treat anything. You should consult a doctor before using this journal. No liability will be accepted for any use or misuse. You use at your own risk and accept all liability.*

BROTHER OR SISTER MEDICAL HISTORY

FULL NAME:

*Disclaimer: This journal is **not** intended to diagnose or treat anything. You should consult a doctor before using this journal. No liability will be accepted for any use or misuse. You use at your own risk and accept all liability.*

Condition	Age at Onset	Treatment	Result
Alzheimer's Disease			
Allergic Rhinitis (Hay fever)			
Anemia			
Anesthesia Problem			
Arthritis			
Asthma			
Birth Defects			
Bleeding Problem			
Cancer, Breast			
Cancer, Colon			
Cancer, Lung			
Cancer, Melanoma			
Cancer, Prostate			
Cancer, Skin			
Cancer, Ovarian			
Cancer (other)			
Depression			
Diabetes, Type 1			
Diabetes, Type 2			
Epilepsy (seizures)			
Eye Conditions			
Glaucoma			
Hearing Problems			
Heart Disease (Coronary Artery or Heart Attack)			
High Cholesterol			

Condition	Age at Onset	Treatment	Result
High Blood Pressure			
Kidney Diseases			
Lupus			
Mental Retardation			
Migraine Headaches			
Miscarriage			
Osteoarthritis			
Osteoporosis			
Rheumatoid Arthritis			
Stroke			
Thyroid Disorders			
Tuberculosis			
Ulcer			
Other:			

OTHER FACTORS

Condition	Age at Onset	Treatment	Result
Alcoholism			
Drug Use			
Obesity			
Smoking			

LIST OF ANY HOSPITALIZATIONS

HOSPITAL: DATE:

REASON:

RESULT:

HOSPITAL: DATE:

REASON:

RESULT:

NOTES

*Disclaimer: This journal is **not** intended to diagnose or treat anything. You should consult a doctor before using this journal. No liability will be accepted for any use or misuse. You use at your own risk and accept all liability.*

BROTHER OR SISTER MEDICAL HISTORY

FULL NAME:

*Disclaimer: This journal is **not** intended to diagnose or treat anything. You should consult a doctor before using this journal. No liability will be accepted for any use or misuse. You use at your own risk and accept all liability.*

Condition	Age at Onset	Treatment	Result
Alzheimer's Disease			
Allergic Rhinitis (Hay fever)			
Anemia			
Anesthesia Problem			
Arthritis			
Asthma			
Birth Defects			
Bleeding Problem			
Cancer, Breast			
Cancer, Colon			
Cancer, Lung			
Cancer, Melanoma			
Cancer, Prostate			
Cancer, Skin			
Cancer, Ovarian			
Cancer (other)			
Depression			
Diabetes, Type 1			
Diabetes, Type 2			
Epilepsy (seizures)			
Eye Conditions			
Glaucoma			
Hearing Problems			
Heart Disease (Coronary Artery or Heart Attack)			
High Cholesterol			

Condition	Age at Onset	Treatment	Result
High Blood Pressure			
Kidney Diseases			
Lupus			
Mental Retardation			
Migraine Headaches			
Miscarriage			
Osteoarthritis			
Osteoporosis			
Rheumatoid Arthritis			
Stroke			
Thyroid Disorders			
Tuberculosis			
Ulcer			
Other:			

OTHER FACTORS

Condition	Age at Onset	Treatment	Result
Alcoholism			
Drug Use			
Obesity			
Smoking			

LIST OF ANY HOSPITALIZATIONS

HOSPITAL: DATE:

REASON:

RESULT:

HOSPITAL: DATE:

REASON:

RESULT:

*Disclaimer: This journal is **not** intended to diagnose or treat anything. You should consult a doctor before using this journal. No liability will be accepted for any use or misuse. You use at your own risk and accept all liability.*

NOTES

*Disclaimer: This journal is **not** intended to diagnose or treat anything. You should consult a doctor before using this journal. No liability will be accepted for any use or misuse. You use at your own risk and accept all liability.*

GRANDFATHER MEDICAL HISTORY

FULL NAME:

*Disclaimer: This journal is **not** intended to diagnose or treat anything. You should consult a doctor before using this journal. No liability will be accepted for any use or misuse. You use at your own risk and accept all liability.*

Condition	Age at Onset	Treatment	Result
Alzheimer's Disease			
Allergic Rhinitis (Hay fever)			
Anemia			
Anesthesia Problem			
Arthritis			
Asthma			
Birth Defects			
Bleeding Problem			
Cancer, Breast			
Cancer, Colon			
Cancer, Lung			
Cancer, Melanoma			
Cancer, Prostate			
Cancer, Skin			
Cancer, Ovarian			
Cancer (other)			
Depression			
Diabetes, Type 1			
Diabetes, Type 2			
Epilepsy (seizures)			
Eye Conditions			
Glaucoma			
Hearing Problems			
Heart Disease (Coronary Artery or Heart Attack)			
High Cholesterol			

Condition	Age at Onset	Treatment	Result
High Blood Pressure			
Kidney Diseases			
Lupus			
Mental Retardation			
Migraine Headaches			
Miscarriage			
Osteoarthritis			
Osteoporosis			
Rheumatoid Arthritis			
Stroke			
Thyroid Disorders			
Tuberculosis			
Ulcer			
Other:			

OTHER FACTORS

Condition	Age at Onset	Treatment	Result
Alcoholism			
Drug Use			
Obesity			
Smoking			

LIST OF ANY HOSPITALIZATIONS

HOSPITAL: DATE:

REASON:

RESULT:

HOSPITAL: DATE:

REASON:

RESULT:

*Disclaimer: This journal is **not** intended to diagnose or treat anything. You should consult a doctor before using this journal. No liability will be accepted for any use or misuse. You use at your own risk and accept all liability.*

NOTES

GRANDMOTHER MEDICAL HISTORY

FULL NAME:

Disclaimer: This journal is ***not*** *intended to diagnose or treat anything. You should consult a doctor before using this journal. No liability will be accepted for any use or misuse. You use at your own risk and accept all liability.*

Condition	Age at Onset	Treatment	Result
Alzheimer's Disease			
Allergic Rhinitis (Hay fever)			
Anemia			
Anesthesia Problem			
Arthritis			
Asthma			
Birth Defects			
Bleeding Problem			
Cancer, Breast			
Cancer, Colon			
Cancer, Lung			
Cancer, Melanoma			
Cancer, Prostate			
Cancer, Skin			
Cancer, Ovarian			
Cancer (other)			
Depression			
Diabetes, Type 1			
Diabetes, Type 2			
Epilepsy (seizures)			
Eye Conditions			
Glaucoma			
Hearing Problems			
Heart Disease (Coronary Artery or Heart Attack)			
High Cholesterol			

Condition	Age at Onset	Treatment	Result
High Blood Pressure			
Kidney Diseases			
Lupus			
Mental Retardation			
Migraine Headaches			
Miscarriage			
Osteoarthritis			
Osteoporosis			
Rheumatoid Arthritis			
Stroke			
Thyroid Disorders			
Tuberculosis			
Ulcer			
Other:			

OTHER FACTORS

Condition	Age at Onset	Treatment	Result
Alcoholism			
Drug Use			
Obesity			
Smoking			

LIST OF ANY HOSPITALIZATIONS

HOSPITAL: DATE:

REASON:

RESULT:

HOSPITAL: DATE:

REASON:

RESULT:

NOTES

*Disclaimer: This journal is **not** intended to diagnose or treat anything. You should consult a doctor before using this journal. No liability will be accepted for any use or misuse. You use at your own risk and accept all liability.*

SPOUSE'S MEDICAL HISTORY

FULL NAME:

*Disclaimer: This journal is **not** intended to diagnose or treat anything. You should consult a doctor before using this journal. No liability will be accepted for any use or misuse. You use at your own risk and accept all liability.*

Condition	Age at Onset	Treatment	Result
Alzheimer's Disease			
Allergic Rhinitis (Hay fever)			
Anemia			
Anesthesia Problem			
Arthritis			
Asthma			
Birth Defects			
Bleeding Problem			
Cancer, Breast			
Cancer, Colon			
Cancer, Lung			
Cancer, Melanoma			
Cancer, Prostate			
Cancer, Skin			
Cancer, Ovarian			
Cancer (other)			
Depression			
Diabetes, Type 1			
Diabetes, Type 2			
Epilepsy (seizures)			
Eye Conditions			
Glaucoma			
Hearing Problems			
Heart Disease (Coronary Artery or Heart Attack)			
High Cholesterol			

Condition	Age at Onset	Treatment	Result
High Blood Pressure			
Kidney Diseases			
Lupus			
Mental Retardation			
Migraine Headaches			
Miscarriage			
Osteoarthritis			
Osteoporosis			
Rheumatoid Arthritis			
Stroke			
Thyroid Disorders			
Tuberculosis			
Ulcer			
Other:			

OTHER FACTORS

Condition	Age at Onset	Treatment	Result
Alcoholism			
Drug Use			
Obesity			
Smoking			

LIST OF ANY HOSPITALIZATIONS

HOSPITAL: DATE:

REASON:

RESULT:

HOSPITAL: DATE:

REASON:

RESULT:

*Disclaimer: This journal is **not** intended to diagnose or treat anything. You should consult a doctor before using this journal. No liability will be accepted for any use or misuse. You use at your own risk and accept all liability.*

NOTES

*Disclaimer: This journal is **not** intended to diagnose or treat anything. You should consult a doctor before using this journal. No liability will be accepted for any use or misuse. You use at your own risk and accept all liability.*

SPOUSE'S FATHER MEDICAL HISTORY

FULL NAME:

*Disclaimer: This journal is **not** intended to diagnose or treat anything. You should consult a doctor before using this journal. No liability will be accepted for any use or misuse. You use at your own risk and accept all liability.*

Condition	Age at Onset	Treatment	Result
Alzheimer's Disease			
Allergic Rhinitis (Hay fever)			
Anemia			
Anesthesia Problem			
Arthritis			
Asthma			
Birth Defects			
Bleeding Problem			
Cancer, Breast			
Cancer, Colon			
Cancer, Lung			
Cancer, Melanoma			
Cancer, Prostate			
Cancer, Skin			
Cancer, Ovarian			
Cancer (other)			
Depression			
Diabetes, Type 1			
Diabetes, Type 2			
Epilepsy (seizures)			
Eye Conditions			
Glaucoma			
Hearing Problems			
Heart Disease (Coronary Artery or Heart Attack)			
High Cholesterol			

Condition	Age at Onset	Treatment	Result
High Blood Pressure			
Kidney Diseases			
Lupus			
Mental Retardation			
Migraine Headaches			
Miscarriage			
Osteoarthritis			
Osteoporosis			
Rheumatoid Arthritis			
Stroke			
Thyroid Disorders			
Tuberculosis			
Ulcer			
Other:			

OTHER FACTORS

Condition	Age at Onset	Treatment	Result
Alcoholism			
Drug Use			
Obesity			
Smoking			

LIST OF ANY HOSPITALIZATIONS

HOSPITAL: DATE:

REASON:

RESULT:

HOSPITAL: DATE:

REASON:

RESULT:

*Disclaimer: This journal is **not** intended to diagnose or treat anything. You should consult a doctor before using this journal. No liability will be accepted for any use or misuse. You use at your own risk and accept all liability.*

NOTES

Disclaimer: This journal is **not** intended to diagnose or treat anything. You should consult a doctor before using this journal. No liability will be accepted for any use or misuse. You use at your own risk and accept all liability.

SPOUSE'S MOTHER MEDICAL HISTORY

FULL NAME:

*Disclaimer: This journal is **not** intended to diagnose or treat anything. You should consult a doctor before using this journal. No liability will be accepted for any use or misuse. You use at your own risk and accept all liability.*

Condition	Age at Onset	Treatment	Result
Alzheimer's Disease			
Allergic Rhinitis (Hay fever)			
Anemia			
Anesthesia Problem			
Arthritis			
Asthma			
Birth Defects			
Bleeding Problem			
Cancer, Breast			
Cancer, Colon			
Cancer, Lung			
Cancer, Melanoma			
Cancer, Prostate			
Cancer, Skin			
Cancer, Ovarian			
Cancer (other)			
Depression			
Diabetes, Type 1			
Diabetes, Type 2			
Epilepsy (seizures)			
Eye Conditions			
Glaucoma			
Hearing Problems			
Heart Disease (Coronary Artery or Heart Attack)			
High Cholesterol			

Condition	Age at Onset	Treatment	Result
High Blood Pressure			
Kidney Diseases			
Lupus			
Mental Retardation			
Migraine Headaches			
Miscarriage			
Osteoarthritis			
Osteoporosis			
Rheumatoid Arthritis			
Stroke			
Thyroid Disorders			
Tuberculosis			
Ulcer			
Other:			

OTHER FACTORS

Condition	Age at Onset	Treatment	Result
Alcoholism			
Drug Use			
Obesity			
Smoking			

LIST OF ANY HOSPITALIZATIONS

HOSPITAL: DATE:

REASON:

RESULT:

HOSPITAL: DATE:

REASON:

RESULT:

*Disclaimer: This journal is **not** intended to diagnose or treat anything. You should consult a doctor before using this journal. No liability will be accepted for any use or misuse. You use at your own risk and accept all liability.*

NOTES

*Disclaimer: This journal is **not** intended to diagnose or treat anything. You should consult a doctor before using this journal. No liability will be accepted for any use or misuse. You use at your own risk and accept all liability.*

SPOUSE'S SIBLING MEDICAL HISTORY

FULL NAME:

*Disclaimer: This journal is **not** intended to diagnose or treat anything. You should consult a doctor before using this journal. No liability will be accepted for any use or misuse. You use at your own risk and accept all liability.*

Condition	Age at Onset	Treatment	Result
Alzheimer's Disease			
Allergic Rhinitis (Hay fever)			
Anemia			
Anesthesia Problem			
Arthritis			
Asthma			
Birth Defects			
Bleeding Problem			
Cancer, Breast			
Cancer, Colon			
Cancer, Lung			
Cancer, Melanoma			
Cancer, Prostate			
Cancer, Skin			
Cancer, Ovarian			
Cancer (other)			
Depression			
Diabetes, Type 1			
Diabetes, Type 2			
Epilepsy (seizures)			
Eye Conditions			
Glaucoma			
Hearing Problems			
Heart Disease (Coronary Artery or Heart Attack)			
High Cholesterol			

Condition	Age at Onset	Treatment	Result
High Blood Pressure			
Kidney Diseases			
Lupus			
Mental Retardation			
Migraine Headaches			
Miscarriage			
Osteoarthritis			
Osteoporosis			
Rheumatoid Arthritis			
Stroke			
Thyroid Disorders			
Tuberculosis			
Ulcer			
Other:			

OTHER FACTORS

Condition	Age at Onset	Treatment	Result
Alcoholism			
Drug Use			
Obesity			
Smoking			

LIST OF ANY HOSPITALIZATIONS

HOSPITAL: DATE:

REASON:

RESULT:

HOSPITAL: DATE:

REASON:

RESULT:

Disclaimer: This journal is ***not*** *intended to diagnose or treat anything. You should consult a doctor before using this journal. No liability will be accepted for any use or misuse. You use at your own risk and accept all liability.*

NOTES

Disclaimer: This journal is ***not*** *intended to diagnose or treat anything. You should consult a doctor before using this journal. No liability will be accepted for any use or misuse. You use at your own risk and accept all liability.*

SPOUSE'S SIBLING MEDICAL HISTORY

FULL NAME:

*Disclaimer: This journal is **not** intended to diagnose or treat anything. You should consult a doctor before using this journal. No liability will be accepted for any use or misuse. You use at your own risk and accept all liability.*

Condition	Age at Onset	Treatment	Result
Alzheimer's Disease			
Allergic Rhinitis (Hay fever)			
Anemia			
Anesthesia Problem			
Arthritis			
Asthma			
Birth Defects			
Bleeding Problem			
Cancer, Breast			
Cancer, Colon			
Cancer, Lung			
Cancer, Melanoma			
Cancer, Prostate			
Cancer, Skin			
Cancer, Ovarian			
Cancer (other)			
Depression			
Diabetes, Type 1			
Diabetes, Type 2			
Epilepsy (seizures)			
Eye Conditions			
Glaucoma			
Hearing Problems			
Heart Disease (Coronary Artery or Heart Attack)			
High Cholesterol			

Condition	Age at Onset	Treatment	Result
High Blood Pressure			
Kidney Diseases			
Lupus			
Mental Retardation			
Migraine Headaches			
Miscarriage			
Osteoarthritis			
Osteoporosis			
Rheumatoid Arthritis			
Stroke			
Thyroid Disorders			
Tuberculosis			
Ulcer			
Other:			

OTHER FACTORS

Condition	Age at Onset	Treatment	Result
Alcoholism			
Drug Use			
Obesity			
Smoking			

LIST OF ANY HOSPITALIZATIONS

HOSPITAL: DATE:

REASON:

RESULT:

HOSPITAL: DATE:

REASON:

RESULT:

*Disclaimer: This journal is **not** intended to diagnose or treat anything. You should consult a doctor before using this journal. No liability will be accepted for any use or misuse. You use at your own risk and accept all liability.*

NOTES

*Disclaimer: This journal is **not** intended to diagnose or treat anything. You should consult a doctor before using this journal. No liability will be accepted for any use or misuse. You use at your own risk and accept all liability.*

SPOUSE'S GRANDFATHER MEDICAL HISTORY

FULL NAME:

*Disclaimer: This journal is **not** intended to diagnose or treat anything. You should consult a doctor before using this journal. No liability will be accepted for any use or misuse. You use at your own risk and accept all liability.*

Condition	Age at Onset	Treatment	Result
Alzheimer's Disease			
Allergic Rhinitis (Hay fever)			
Anemia			
Anesthesia Problem			
Arthritis			
Asthma			
Birth Defects			
Bleeding Problem			
Cancer, Breast			
Cancer, Colon			
Cancer, Lung			
Cancer, Melanoma			
Cancer, Prostate			
Cancer, Skin			
Cancer, Ovarian			
Cancer (other)			
Depression			
Diabetes, Type 1			
Diabetes, Type 2			
Epilepsy (seizures)			
Eye Conditions			
Glaucoma			
Hearing Problems			
Heart Disease (Coronary Artery or Heart Attack)			
High Cholesterol			

Condition	Age at Onset	Treatment	Result
High Blood Pressure			
Kidney Diseases			
Lupus			
Mental Retardation			
Migraine Headaches			
Miscarriage			
Osteoarthritis			
Osteoporosis			
Rheumatoid Arthritis			
Stroke			
Thyroid Disorders			
Tuberculosis			
Ulcer			
Other:			

OTHER FACTORS

Condition	Age at Onset	Treatment	Result
Alcoholism			
Drug Use			
Obesity			
Smoking			

LIST OF ANY HOSPITALIZATIONS

HOSPITAL: DATE:

REASON:

RESULT:

HOSPITAL: DATE:

REASON:

RESULT:

*Disclaimer: This journal is **not** intended to diagnose or treat anything. You should consult a doctor before using this journal. No liability will be accepted for any use or misuse. You use at your own risk and accept all liability.*

NOTES

SPOUSE'S GRANDMOTHER MEDICAL HISTORY

FULL NAME:

*Disclaimer: This journal is **not** intended to diagnose or treat anything. You should consult a doctor before using this journal. No liability will be accepted for any use or misuse. You use at your own risk and accept all liability.*

Condition	Age at Onset	Treatment	Result
Alzheimer's Disease			
Allergic Rhinitis (Hay fever)			
Anemia			
Anesthesia Problem			
Arthritis			
Asthma			
Birth Defects			
Bleeding Problem			
Cancer, Breast			
Cancer, Colon			
Cancer, Lung			
Cancer, Melanoma			
Cancer, Prostate			
Cancer, Skin			
Cancer, Ovarian			
Cancer (other)			
Depression			
Diabetes, Type 1			
Diabetes, Type 2			
Epilepsy (seizures)			
Eye Conditions			
Glaucoma			
Hearing Problems			
Heart Disease (Coronary Artery or Heart Attack)			
High Cholesterol			

Condition	Age at Onset	Treatment	Result
High Blood Pressure			
Kidney Diseases			
Lupus			
Mental Retardation			
Migraine Headaches			
Miscarriage			
Osteoarthritis			
Osteoporosis			
Rheumatoid Arthritis			
Stroke			
Thyroid Disorders			
Tuberculosis			
Ulcer			
Other:			

OTHER FACTORS

Condition	Age at Onset	Treatment	Result
Alcoholism			
Drug Use			
Obesity			
Smoking			

LIST OF ANY HOSPITALIZATIONS

HOSPITAL: DATE:

REASON:

RESULT:

HOSPITAL: DATE:

REASON:

RESULT:

*Disclaimer: This journal is **not** intended to diagnose or treat anything. You should consult a doctor before using this journal. No liability will be accepted for any use or misuse. You use at your own risk and accept all liability.*

YOUR VACCINE RECORDS

FULL NAME	BIRTHDATE

VACCINE	TYPE OF VACCINE	DATE GIVEN MO/DA/YR	HEATHCARE PROFESSIONAL OR CLINIC	DATE NEXT DOSE DUE
Hepatitis B6				
Diphtheria, Tetanus, Pertussis6				
Haemophilus influenzae type b6				
Polio6				

*Disclaimer: This journal is **not** intended to diagnose or treat anything. You should consult a doctor before using this journal. No liability will be accepted for any use or misuse. You use at your own risk and accept all liability.*

YOUR VACCINE RECORDS

FULL NAME	BIRTHDATE

VACCINE	TYPE OF VACCINE	DATE GIVEN MO/DA/YR	HEATHCARE PROFESSIONAL OR CLINIC	DATE NEXT DOSE DUE
Pneumococcal				
Rotavirus				
Measles, Mumps, Rubella6				
Varicella6				
Hepatitis A				
Meningococcal				
Human papillomavirus				

YOUR VACCINE RECORDS

FULL NAME	BIRTHDATE

VACCINE	TYPE OF VACCINE	DATE GIVEN MO/DA/YR	HEATHCARE PROFESSIONAL OR CLINIC	DATE NEXT DOSE DUE
Influenza				
Other				

*Disclaimer: This journal is **not** intended to diagnose or treat anything. You should consult a doctor before using this journal. No liability will be accepted for any use or misuse. You use at your own risk and accept all liability.*

SPOUSE'S VACCINE RECORDS

FULL NAME	BIRTHDATE

VACCINE	TYPE OF VACCINE	DATE GIVEN MO/DA/YR	HEATHCARE PROFESSIONAL OR CLINIC	DATE NEXT DOSE DUE
Hepatitis B6				
Diphtheria, Tetanus, Pertussis6				
Haemophilus influenzae type b6				
Polio6				

SPOUSE'S VACCINE RECORDS

FULL NAME	BIRTHDATE

VACCINE	TYPE OF VACCINE	DATE GIVEN MO/DA/YR	HEATHCARE PROFESSIONAL OR CLINIC	DATE NEXT DOSE DUE
Pneumococcal				
Rotavirus				
Measles, Mumps, Rubella6				
Varicella6				
Hepatitis A				
Meningococcal				
Human papillomavirus				

SPOUSE'S VACCINE RECORDS

FULL NAME	BIRTHDATE

VACCINE	TYPE OF VACCINE	DATE GIVEN MO/DA/YR	HEATHCARE PROFESSIONAL OR CLINIC	DATE NEXT DOSE DUE
Influenza				
Other				

*Disclaimer: This journal is **not** intended to diagnose or treat anything. You should consult a doctor before using this journal. No liability will be accepted for any use or misuse. You use at your own risk and accept all liability.*

CHILD'S VACCINE RECORDS

FULL NAME	BIRTHDATE

VACCINE	TYPE OF VACCINE	DATE GIVEN MO/DA/YR	HEATHCARE PROFESSIONAL OR CLINIC	DATE NEXT DOSE DUE
Hepatitis B6				
Diphtheria, Tetanus, Pertussis6				
Haemophilus influenzae type b6				
Polio6				

CHILD'S VACCINE RECORDS

FULL NAME	BIRTHDATE

VACCINE	TYPE OF VACCINE	DATE GIVEN MO/DA/YR	HEATHCARE PROFESSIONAL OR CLINIC	DATE NEXT DOSE DUE
Pneumococcal				
Rotavirus				
Measles, Mumps, Rubella6				
Varicella6				
Hepatitis A				
Meningococcal				
Human papillomavirus				

CHILD'S VACCINE RECORDS

FULL NAME	BIRTHDATE

VACCINE	TYPE OF VACCINE	DATE GIVEN MO/DA/YR	HEATHCARE PROFESSIONAL OR CLINIC	DATE NEXT DOSE DUE
Influenza				
Other				

*Disclaimer: This journal is **not** intended to diagnose or treat anything. You should consult a doctor before using this journal. No liability will be accepted for any use or misuse. You use at your own risk and accept all liability.*

CHILD'S VACCINE RECORDS

FULL NAME	BIRTHDATE

VACCINE	TYPE OF VACCINE	DATE GIVEN MO/DA/YR	HEATHCARE PROFESSIONAL OR CLINIC	DATE NEXT DOSE DUE
Hepatitis B[6]				
Diphtheria, Tetanus, Pertussis[6]				
Haemophilus influenzae type b[6]				
Polio[6]				

CHILD'S VACCINE RECORDS

FULL NAME	BIRTHDATE

VACCINE	TYPE OF VACCINE	DATE GIVEN MO/DA/YR	HEATHCARE PROFESSIONAL OR CLINIC	DATE NEXT DOSE DUE
Pneumococcal				
Rotavirus				
Measles, Mumps, Rubella6				
Varicella6				
Hepatitis A				
Meningococcal				
Human papillomavirus				

CHILD'S VACCINE RECORDS

FULL NAME	BIRTHDATE

VACCINE	TYPE OF VACCINE	DATE GIVEN MO/DA/YR	HEATHCARE PROFESSIONAL OR CLINIC	DATE NEXT DOSE DUE
Influenza				
Other				

*Disclaimer: This journal is **not** intended to diagnose or treat anything. You should consult a doctor before using this journal. No liability will be accepted for any use or misuse. You use at your own risk and accept all liability.*

CHILD'S VACCINE RECORDS

FULL NAME	BIRTHDATE

VACCINE	TYPE OF VACCINE	DATE GIVEN MO/DA/YR	HEATHCARE PROFESSIONAL OR CLINIC	DATE NEXT DOSE DUE
Hepatitis B6				
Diphtheria, Tetanus, Pertussis6				
Haemophilus influenzae type b6				
Polio6				

CHILD'S VACCINE RECORDS

FULL NAME	BIRTHDATE

VACCINE	TYPE OF VACCINE	DATE GIVEN MO/DA/YR	HEATHCARE PROFESSIONAL OR CLINIC	DATE NEXT DOSE DUE
Pneumococcal				
Rotavirus				
Measles, Mumps, Rubella6				
Varicella6				
Hepatitis A				
Meningococcal				
Human papillomavirus				

CHILD'S VACCINE RECORDS

FULL NAME	BIRTHDATE

VACCINE	TYPE OF VACCINE	DATE GIVEN MO/DA/YR	HEATHCARE PROFESSIONAL OR CLINIC	DATE NEXT DOSE DUE
Influenza				
Other				

*Disclaimer: This journal is **not** intended to diagnose or treat anything. You should consult a doctor before using this journal. No liability will be accepted for any use or misuse. You use at your own risk and accept all liability.*

LABORATORY TESTS

FULL NAME	BIRTHDATE

DATE	TEST	RESULTS

LABORATORY TESTS

FULL NAME	BIRTHDATE

DATE	TEST	RESULTS

LABORATORY TESTS

FULL NAME	BIRTHDATE

DATE	TEST	RESULTS

LABORATORY TESTS

FULL NAME	BIRTHDATE

DATE	TEST	RESULTS

LABORATORY TESTS

FULL NAME	BIRTHDATE

DATE	TEST	RESULTS

LABORATORY TESTS

FULL NAME	BIRTHDATE

DATE	TEST	RESULTS

LABORATORY TESTS

FULL NAME	BIRTHDATE

DATE	TEST	RESULTS

LABORATORY TESTS

FULL NAME	BIRTHDATE

DATE	TEST	RESULTS

LABORATORY TESTS

FULL NAME	BIRTHDATE

DATE	TEST	RESULTS

LABORATORY TESTS

FULL NAME	BIRTHDATE

DATE	TEST	RESULTS

LABORATORY TESTS

FULL NAME	BIRTHDATE

DATE	TEST	RESULTS

HEIGHT & WEIGHT

FULL NAME	BIRTHDATE

DATE	HEIGHT	WEIGHT

HEIGHT & WEIGHT

FULL NAME	BIRTHDATE

DATE	HEIGHT	WEIGHT

HEIGHT & WEIGHT

FULL NAME	BIRTHDATE

DATE	HEIGHT	WEIGHT

HEIGHT & WEIGHT

FULL NAME	BIRTHDATE

DATE	HEIGHT	WEIGHT

HEIGHT & WEIGHT

FULL NAME	BIRTHDATE

DATE	HEIGHT	WEIGHT

DENTAL RECORDS

FULL NAME	BIRTHDATE

DATE	DENTIST NAME	PROCEDURE	RESULT

NOTES

*Disclaimer: This journal is **not** intended to diagnose or treat anything. You should consult a doctor before using this journal. No liability will be accepted for any use or misuse. You use at your own risk and accept all liability.*

DENTAL RECORDS

FULL NAME	BIRTHDATE

DATE	DENTIST NAME	PROCEDURE	RESULT

NOTES

*Disclaimer: This journal is **not** intended to diagnose or treat anything. You should consult a doctor before using this journal. No liability will be accepted for any use or misuse. You use at your own risk and accept all liability.*

DENTAL RECORDS

FULL NAME	BIRTHDATE

DATE	DENTIST NAME	PROCEDURE	RESULT

NOTES

DENTAL RECORDS

FULL NAME	BIRTHDATE

DATE	DENTIST NAME	PROCEDURE	RESULT

NOTES

*Disclaimer: This journal is **not** intended to diagnose or treat anything. You should consult a doctor before using this journal. No liability will be accepted for any use or misuse. You use at your own risk and accept all liability.*

DENTAL RECORDS

FULL NAME	BIRTHDATE

DATE	DENTIST NAME	PROCEDURE	RESULT

VISION RECORDS

FULL NAME	BIRTHDATE

DATE	OPTICAL NAME	PROCEDURE	RESULT

VISION RECORDS

FULL NAME	BIRTHDATE

DATE	OPTICAL NAME	PROCEDURE	RESULT

VISION RECORDS

FULL NAME	BIRTHDATE

DATE	OPTICAL NAME	PROCEDURE	RESULT

VISION RECORDS

FULL NAME	BIRTHDATE

DATE	OPTICAL NAME	PROCEDURE	RESULT

VISION RECORDS

FULL NAME	BIRTHDATE

DATE	OPTICAL NAME	PROCEDURE	RESULT

X-RAY, SCAN RECORDS

FULL NAME	BIRTHDATE

DATE	PROCEDURE	RESULT

NOTES

*Disclaimer: This journal is **not** intended to diagnose or treat anything. You should consult a doctor before using this journal. No liability will be accepted for any use or misuse. You use at your own risk and accept all liability.*

X-RAY, SCAN RECORDS

FULL NAME	BIRTHDATE

DATE	PROCEDURE	RESULT

NOTES

*Disclaimer: This journal is **not** intended to diagnose or treat anything. You should consult a doctor before using this journal. No liability will be accepted for any use or misuse. You use at your own risk and accept all liability.*

X-RAY, SCAN RECORDS

FULL NAME	BIRTHDATE

DATE	PROCEDURE	RESULT

NOTES

*Disclaimer: This journal is **not** intended to diagnose or treat anything. You should consult a doctor before using this journal. No liability will be accepted for any use or misuse. You use at your own risk and accept all liability.*

X-RAY, SCAN RECORDS

FULL NAME	BIRTHDATE

DATE	PROCEDURE	RESULT

NOTES

X-RAY, SCAN RECORDS

FULL NAME	BIRTHDATE

DATE	PROCEDURE	RESULT

APPOINTMENT NOTES / QUESTIONS FOR DOCTOR

FULL NAME	BIRTHDATE

DATE	QUESTION	DOCTORS ANSWER

NOTES

APPOINTMENT NOTES / QUESTIONS FOR DOCTOR

FULL NAME	BIRTHDATE

DATE	QUESTION	DOCTORS ANSWER

NOTES

*Disclaimer: This journal is **not** intended to diagnose or treat anything. You should consult a doctor before using this journal. No liability will be accepted for any use or misuse. You use at your own risk and accept all liability.*

APPOINTMENT NOTES / QUESTIONS FOR DOCTOR

FULL NAME	BIRTHDATE

DATE	QUESTION	DOCTORS ANSWER

NOTES

*Disclaimer: This journal is **not** intended to diagnose or treat anything. You should consult a doctor before using this journal. No liability will be accepted for any use or misuse. You use at your own risk and accept all liability.*

APPOINTMENT NOTES / QUESTIONS FOR DOCTOR

FULL NAME	BIRTHDATE

DATE	QUESTION	DOCTORS ANSWER

NOTES

*Disclaimer: This journal is **not** intended to diagnose or treat anything. You should consult a doctor before using this journal. No liability will be accepted for any use or misuse. You use at your own risk and accept all liability.*

APPOINTMENT NOTES / QUESTIONS FOR DOCTOR

FULL NAME	BIRTHDATE

DATE	QUESTION	DOCTORS ANSWER

NOTES

*Disclaimer: This journal is **not** intended to diagnose or treat anything. You should consult a doctor before using this journal. No liability will be accepted for any use or misuse. You use at your own risk and accept all liability.*

APPOINTMENT NOTES / QUESTIONS FOR DOCTOR

FULL NAME	BIRTHDATE

DATE	QUESTION	DOCTORS ANSWER

NOTES

Disclaimer: This journal is ***not*** *intended to diagnose or treat anything. You should consult a doctor before using this journal. No liability will be accepted for any use or misuse. You use at your own risk and accept all liability.*

APPOINTMENT NOTES / QUESTIONS FOR DOCTOR

FULL NAME	BIRTHDATE

DATE	QUESTION	DOCTORS ANSWER

NOTES

APPOINTMENT NOTES / QUESTIONS FOR DOCTOR

FULL NAME	BIRTHDATE

DATE	QUESTION	DOCTORS ANSWER

NOTES

*Disclaimer: This journal is **not** intended to diagnose or treat anything. You should consult a doctor before using this journal. No liability will be accepted for any use or misuse. You use at your own risk and accept all liability.*

APPOINTMENT NOTES / QUESTIONS FOR DOCTOR

FULL NAME	BIRTHDATE

DATE	QUESTION	DOCTORS ANSWER

NOTES

*Disclaimer: This journal is **not** intended to diagnose or treat anything. You should consult a doctor before using this journal. No liability will be accepted for any use or misuse. You use at your own risk and accept all liability.*

APPOINTMENT NOTES / QUESTIONS FOR DOCTOR

FULL NAME	BIRTHDATE

DATE	QUESTION	DOCTORS ANSWER

DOCTORS YOU HAVE SEEN

FULL NAME	BIRTHDATE

DATE	DOCTORS INFORMATION	CONDITION

DOCTORS YOU HAVE SEEN

FULL NAME	BIRTHDATE

DATE	DOCTORS INFORMATION	CONDITION

DOCTORS YOU HAVE SEEN

FULL NAME	BIRTHDATE

DATE	DOCTORS INFORMATION	CONDITION

DOCTORS YOU HAVE SEEN

FULL NAME	BIRTHDATE

DATE	DOCTORS INFORMATION	CONDITION

DOCTORS YOU HAVE SEEN

FULL NAME	BIRTHDATE

DATE	DOCTORS INFORMATION	CONDITION

DOCTORS YOU HAVE SEEN

FULL NAME	BIRTHDATE

DATE	DOCTORS INFORMATION	CONDITION

DOCTORS YOU HAVE SEEN

FULL NAME	BIRTHDATE

DATE	DOCTORS INFORMATION	CONDITION

DOCTORS YOU HAVE SEEN

FULL NAME	BIRTHDATE

DATE	DOCTORS INFORMATION	CONDITION

DOCTORS YOU HAVE SEEN

FULL NAME	BIRTHDATE

DATE	DOCTORS INFORMATION	CONDITION

DOCTORS YOU HAVE SEEN

FULL NAME	BIRTHDATE

DATE	DOCTORS INFORMATION	CONDITION

DOCTORS YOU HAVE SEEN

FULL NAME	BIRTHDATE

DATE	DOCTORS INFORMATION	CONDITION

DOCTORS YOU HAVE SEEN

FULL NAME	BIRTHDATE

DATE	DOCTORS INFORMATION	CONDITION

MEDICATION RECORDS

FULL NAME	BIRTHDATE

DATE	NAME OF MEDICATON	TIME TAKEN	AMOUNT TAKEN

NOTES

*Disclaimer: This journal is **not** intended to diagnose or treat anything. You should consult a doctor before using this journal. No liability will be accepted for any use or misuse. You use at your own risk and accept all liability.*

MEDICATION RECORDS

FULL NAME	BIRTHDATE

DATE	NAME OF MEDICATON	TIME TAKEN	AMOUNT TAKEN

NOTES

MEDICATION RECORDS

FULL NAME	BIRTHDATE

DATE	NAME OF MEDICATON	TIME TAKEN	AMOUNT TAKEN

NOTES

*Disclaimer: This journal is **not** intended to diagnose or treat anything. You should consult a doctor before using this journal. No liability will be accepted for any use or misuse. You use at your own risk and accept all liability.*

MEDICATION RECORDS

FULL NAME	BIRTHDATE

DATE	NAME OF MEDICATON	TIME TAKEN	AMOUNT TAKEN

NOTES

*Disclaimer: This journal is **not** intended to diagnose or treat anything. You should consult a doctor before using this journal. No liability will be accepted for any use or misuse. You use at your own risk and accept all liability.*

MEDICATION RECORDS

FULL NAME	BIRTHDATE

DATE	NAME OF MEDICATON	TIME TAKEN	AMOUNT TAKEN

NOTES

*Disclaimer: This journal is **not** intended to diagnose or treat anything. You should consult a doctor before using this journal. No liability will be accepted for any use or misuse. You use at your own risk and accept all liability.*

MEDICATION RECORDS

FULL NAME	BIRTHDATE

DATE	NAME OF MEDICATON	TIME TAKEN	AMOUNT TAKEN

NOTES

*Disclaimer: This journal is **not** intended to diagnose or treat anything. You should consult a doctor before using this journal. No liability will be accepted for any use or misuse. You use at your own risk and accept all liability.*

MEDICATION RECORDS

FULL NAME	BIRTHDATE

DATE	NAME OF MEDICATON	TIME TAKEN	AMOUNT TAKEN

NOTES

*Disclaimer: This journal is **not** intended to diagnose or treat anything. You should consult a doctor before using this journal. No liability will be accepted for any use or misuse. You use at your own risk and accept all liability.*

MEDICATION RECORDS

FULL NAME	BIRTHDATE

DATE	NAME OF MEDICATON	TIME TAKEN	AMOUNT TAKEN

NOTES

*Disclaimer: This journal is **not** intended to diagnose or treat anything. You should consult a doctor before using this journal. No liability will be accepted for any use or misuse. You use at your own risk and accept all liability.*

MEDICATION RECORDS

FULL NAME	BIRTHDATE

DATE	NAME OF MEDICATON	TIME TAKEN	AMOUNT TAKEN

NOTES

Disclaimer: This journal is ***not*** *intended to diagnose or treat anything. You should consult a doctor before using this journal. No liability will be accepted for any use or misuse. You use at your own risk and accept all liability.*

MEDICATION RECORDS

FULL NAME	BIRTHDATE

DATE	NAME OF MEDICATON	TIME TAKEN	AMOUNT TAKEN

NOTES

Disclaimer: *This journal is* ***not*** *intended to diagnose or treat anything. You should consult a doctor before using this journal. No liability will be accepted for any use or misuse. You use at your own risk and accept all liability.*

MEDICATION RECORDS

FULL NAME	BIRTHDATE

DATE	NAME OF MEDICATON	TIME TAKEN	AMOUNT TAKEN

MEDICATION RECORDS

FULL NAME	BIRTHDATE

DATE	NAME OF MEDICATON	TIME TAKEN	AMOUNT TAKEN

MEDICATION RECORDS

FULL NAME	BIRTHDATE

DATE	NAME OF MEDICATON	TIME TAKEN	AMOUNT TAKEN

MEDICATION RECORDS

FULL NAME	BIRTHDATE

DATE	NAME OF MEDICATON	TIME TAKEN	AMOUNT TAKEN

MEDICATION RECORDS

FULL NAME	BIRTHDATE

DATE	NAME OF MEDICATON	TIME TAKEN	AMOUNT TAKEN

MEDICATION RECORDS

FULL NAME	BIRTHDATE

DATE	NAME OF MEDICATON	TIME TAKEN	AMOUNT TAKEN

MEDICATION RECORDS

FULL NAME	BIRTHDATE

DATE	NAME OF MEDICATON	TIME TAKEN	AMOUNT TAKEN

MEDICATION RECORDS

FULL NAME	BIRTHDATE

DATE	NAME OF MEDICATON	TIME TAKEN	AMOUNT TAKEN

MEDICATION RECORDS

FULL NAME	BIRTHDATE

DATE	NAME OF MEDICATON	TIME TAKEN	AMOUNT TAKEN

MEDICATION RECORDS

FULL NAME	BIRTHDATE

DATE	NAME OF MEDICATON	TIME TAKEN	AMOUNT TAKEN

SURGERY RECORDS

FULL NAME	BIRTHDATE

DATE	DOCTOR	SURGERY TYPE

SURGERY RECORDS

FULL NAME	BIRTHDATE

DATE	DOCTOR	SURGERY TYPE

SURGERY RECORDS

FULL NAME	BIRTHDATE

DATE	DOCTOR	SURGERY TYPE

SURGERY RECORDS

FULL NAME	BIRTHDATE

DATE	DOCTOR	SURGERY TYPE

SURGERY RECORDS

FULL NAME	BIRTHDATE

DATE	DOCTOR	SURGERY TYPE

SURGERY RECORDS

FULL NAME	BIRTHDATE

DATE	DOCTOR	SURGERY TYPE

SURGERY RECORDS

FULL NAME	BIRTHDATE

DATE	DOCTOR	SURGERY TYPE

ENT RECORDS

FULL NAME	BIRTHDATE

DATE	DOCTOR	RESULTS

ENT RECORDS

FULL NAME	BIRTHDATE

DATE	DOCTOR	RESULTS

ENT RECORDS

FULL NAME	BIRTHDATE

DATE	DOCTOR	RESULTS

ENT RECORDS

FULL NAME	BIRTHDATE

DATE	DOCTOR	RESULTS

ENT RECORDS

FULL NAME	BIRTHDATE

DATE	DOCTOR	RESULTS

SYMPTOM RECORDS

FULL NAME	BIRTHDATE

DATE	SYMPTOM	ACTION TAKEN

NOTES

*Disclaimer: This journal is **not** intended to diagnose or treat anything. You should consult a doctor before using this journal. No liability will be accepted for any use or misuse. You use at your own risk and accept all liability.*

SYMPTOM RECORDS

FULL NAME	BIRTHDATE

DATE	SYMPTOM	ACTION TAKEN

NOTES

Disclaimer: This journal is ***not*** *intended to diagnose or treat anything. You should consult a doctor before using this journal. No liability will be accepted for any use or misuse. You use at your own risk and accept all liability.*

SYMPTOM RECORDS

FULL NAME	BIRTHDATE

DATE	SYMPTOM	ACTION TAKEN

SYMPTOM RECORDS

FULL NAME	BIRTHDATE

DATE	SYMPTOM	ACTION TAKEN

SYMPTOM RECORDS

FULL NAME	BIRTHDATE

DATE	SYMPTOM	ACTION TAKEN

SYMPTOM RECORDS

FULL NAME	BIRTHDATE

DATE	SYMPTOM	ACTION TAKEN

SYMPTOM RECORDS

FULL NAME	BIRTHDATE

DATE	SYMPTOM	ACTION TAKEN

SYMPTOM RECORDS

FULL NAME	BIRTHDATE

DATE	SYMPTOM	ACTION TAKEN

SYMPTOM RECORDS

FULL NAME	BIRTHDATE

DATE	SYMPTOM	ACTION TAKEN

SYMPTOM RECORDS

FULL NAME	BIRTHDATE

DATE	SYMPTOM	ACTION TAKEN

SYMPTOM RECORDS

FULL NAME	BIRTHDATE

DATE	SYMPTOM	ACTION TAKEN

Made in the USA
Monee, IL
04 November 2026

67383083R00115